Child Growth And Hair Care Book

Olatundun Solomon

olatundunsolomon@gmail.com

The growth of the
child is very
important. Taking
care of the child in
order to have normal
growth is important.
Normal growth and
development of the
child is necessary. The
human body has cells,
tissues, organs and
systems. All needs to

function normally.
The human body has
eye, ear, mouth, nose,
brain in the head,
heart in inside the
body in the chest
region, kidneys, liver,
spleen, bladder,
intestines, stomach
and lungs are in the
body. The child did
not need any thing

that can alter normal
growth.

These are ways care
of a child for normal
growth can be done.

(1). The Child Should
Eat Protein Food.

Protein food is
important for the
child to grow. Protein
food makes the body
grow and develop.
Examples, of protein

foods are: Titus fish,
sardine fish, beans,
egg, chicken, turkey,
peanut and milk.

There are other foods
that should also be
eaten with protein
food for the body to
be healthy. These are:

(2). Carbohydrates:
Carbohydrate is
energy food.
Examples are:
potatoes, yam, wheat,
sorghum, rice and
maize. Carbohydrate
food makes the child
to have energy.

(3). Vitamins And
Minerals: Vitamins

and minerals makes the body to have immunity. This helps the body to fight against diseases. Examples of foods that has vitamins and minerals are: Cabbage, lettuce, apple, watermelon, pawpaw, orange, cucumber, pineapple,

tomatoes, pepper,
onions, avocados,
pumpkin, eggplant
and mango.

(4). Water:

Drinking clean water
is very important. It
helps in the digestion
of food. It helps in the

hydration of the body. It prevent dehydration. Bathing with clean water and soap makes the body to be clean. This prevent disease causing microorganisms. This can prevent diseases that can alter skin growth.

(5). Oil:

Oil makes the joints
of the body to be
lubricated. This
makes arthritis to be
prevented. This
makes the joints of
the body to grow well

in children. Oily foods makes the body to have warmth. Examples of oily foods are peanut, cashew nut, sardine fish, avocados and vegetable oil.

(6). Smoking Of
Cigarettes Should Not
Be Done.

Cigarettes smoking
can cause lung cancer.
This can make the
lungs not to grow
well. Cigarettes
smoking can also
affect the liver
function negatively.
Cigarettes smoking

can affect the appearance of the lips and soles of the feet negatively.

(7). Take Children To The Hospital To Have Good Care.

Children should be taken to the hospital in order to have good care. Normal prescription of drugs should be taken in order to have normal care.

(8). The child should have good sleep in order to have good growth of the body.

(9). The Child Should
Have Exercise.

Exercise makes the
body grow well and
to be healthy.

Hair is part of the
human body. The hair
needs a lot of care.
The infection of the
hair can lead to
infection of other
parts of the body.
These are ways you
can take care of the
hair.

1. Oily food: Oily
foods can be eaten
and this can make the
hair to have oil. This
can make the hair not
to break. This can
make the skin of the
body to look glossy
and also the hair to
look glossy. Examples

of oily foods are:
cashew nuts, peanuts,
sardine fish,
avocadoes, soya
beans oil and
vegetable oil.

2. Fruits: Fruits has
vitamins and minerals.
When fruits are eaten,
such as apple,
pineapple, orange,

mango and papaya. It makes the hair to be well nourished. This makes the hair to be healthy.

3. Vegetables: Vegetables has vitamins and minerals. When vegetables such as cabbage, cucumber and lettuce

are eaten it makes the hair to be well nourished. This makes the hair to be healthy.

4. Protein: Protein makes the body to grow. This makes the hair to grow. Protein foods are Titus fish, sardine fish, beans,

peanut, milk, egg,
beef, turkey and
chicken.

5. Bath: Taking bath
with soap and water
makes the hair to be
clean and healthy.

6. Water: Drinking
clean water hydrate

the body. The hair
can be healthy by
drinking clean water.
This can make the
hair not to be dry or
break.

7. Exercise: Exercise
makes the body to be
healthy. This makes
the hair to be healthy.

8. Sleep: Sleeping enough refreshes the body. This makes the hair to be healthy.

9. Chefs and also females should not use dirty scarfs to cover the hair. Dirty

scarfs can lead to hair

infections and also

skin infections.